Weight Management

by

Gilbert B. Bradham, M. D.

Table of Contents

Chapter I

Weight Management

Weight management is designed for those persons whose weight exceeds an optimal body composition because of the accumulated storage of fat. This issue is of serious importance because accumulation of excessive fat is associated with diabetes, cancer, stroke, loss of energy, social and emotional problems, and the necessity to carry the accumulated fat around all day long.

The Weight Management methods explained in this book have been proven by management of thousands of persons. We have found a 100% success rate among persons who followed our advice. Our methods have been applied to hundreds of persons who have failed in numerous current programs including Jennie Craig, Weight Watchers, Atkins, South Beach, and the Zone. The major differences between our methods and others are that we offer more and better information, liberal use of appetite suppressants, and frequent contact with expertise in weight management.

The cornerstone of weight management is the information that allows a thorough comprehension of why a person has gained too much weight, the potential harm that can be caused by excessive weight, and frequent guidance by an experienced health professional.

The management of weight is management of food. Human beings eat only three kinds of food: carbohydrate, fat and protein. Protein forms the structure of the body while carbohydrate and fat are burned (oxidized) to provide energy to do work. When too much fat is ingested, it is stored. When too much carbohydrate is ingested, it is stored as fat. Weight management, then, is simply a knowledgeable plan to limit fat and carbohydrate to the extent that excessive storage does not occur.

Weight management, though conceptually simple, is not easy. Persons who were allowed to eat anything and as much as they wanted as children, have gained satisfaction from food in many ways. Cooking food is interesting. Look at the number of books in any bookstore devoted to how to prepare and cook the same foods. Notice the number of catalogs selling cookware, the same old pots and pans, and the hundreds of knives and knife sharpeners to cut food. Beyond the expensive stoves, refrigerators and freezers in the kitchen, millions of grills lay waiting in the backyard.

Food looks good, tastes good and is satiating. Food replaces boredom, offsets stress, communicates messages and is the backbone of social intercourse. Food is a staple of all religions (the Lord's Supper), ammunition for the troops, and the entrée to sex (with wine).

Carbohydrate and fat are necessary to provide energy for work to maintain the body and energy by which to work on our environment. Energy is even necessary to attain more energy. The culprit is excess. Weight management is a method of learning how much energy is necessary and how to curb excess.

To begin to understand this process it is well to first understand how the bodies of men and women are composed.

Chapter II

Normal Body Composition

The human body is composed of muscle, fat, bone and material we will call "other." Brain, skin, gut, and other material comprise this "other" category.

A young, healthy, normal (average) male is 15% fat, 45% muscle, 15% bone and 25% other.

A young, healthy, normal (average) female is 27% fat, 36% muscle, 12% bone and 25% other.

The female proportionally has more fat, less muscle, less bone and the same other.

These values were obtained with careful research on thousands of individuals.[1]

Fat exists in two forms: essential fat and storage fat. Essential fat is stored in bone marrow, heart, liver, lungs, kidney, skin, and the nervous system. This fat is required for normal physiological function. In the female some of the essential fat is sex-specific, characteristic of breast, abdominal, hips, buttocks and extremity structure.

The other depot of fat is storage fat located in various organs, abdomen, and beneath the skin. Storage fat is nutritional fat used to burn and provide energy. It is storage fat which becomes excessive if not used at a rate needed to provide internal and external work.

It is conceptually easy to remember that men should have less than 20% total fat and that women should have less than 30% total fat.

For example, if a man weighs 190 pounds and is 20% fat then he is carrying 36 pounds of fat. If a women weights 180 pounds and is 30% fat she is carrying 54 pounds of fat. When either gains 20 extra pounds it is similar to wearing a knapsack with 20 pounds of bricks, all the time, to church, the bathroom, while shopping or socializing.

In understanding the normal (average) body composition it becomes imperative that height-weight tables are only approximations. As an

---

1   *Exercise Physiology, 3rd Edition,* McArdle, Katch, and Katch

example, consider two 180 pound men. One is a professional athlete whose fat content is only 10% instead of 15% and his muscle mass is 50% instead of 45%. The second man is a couch potato with a fat content of 30% and a muscle mass of 30%. Both weigh the same but one is muscle and the other is fat.

Put another way, suppose a woman wants to lose weight primarily by exercising. She goes to the gym and begins weight training. She builds 10 lbs of muscle and loses 10 lbs of fat. She is now stronger, has more energy, feels better, but is disappointed that she hasn't lost weight.

It is, therefore, important to realize that while exercise is great for body, mind and spirit, exercise alone is not the effective way to lose fat. The effective way to lose fat is to curb excessive food intake. This book is devoted to that subject, but first it is important to review more about the composition of foods.

Chapter III

Foods

All of our foods can be categorized as carbohydrates, fats or proteins.

Carbohydrates are combinations of carbon and water that form sugars. Carbohydrates are sugars. The most common form of sugar is sucrose that is derived from sugarcane, sugar beets, maple syrup and honey. Sucrose is table sugar and is the most common constituent of all processed foods. Lactose is milk sugar and maltose occurs in malt products and germinating cereal. Fructose is the prevailing sugar in fruit. Carbohydrate is the general name for sugars and comprises most of what is found in the center of grocery stores. Meat, eggs, milk and vegetables are generally on the periphery. When on a low carbohydrate diet, stay out of the middle of grocery stores.

All carbohydrates, whether from bread, pasta, potato, corn, wheat or fruit, break down in the human body to a simple sugar, glucose. Glucose is then used for energy, stored as glycogen or stored as fat. Glucose is used to provide energy. It does this by a complex reaction that liberates high energy molecules called ATP (adenosine triphosphate), ADP (adenosine diphosphate) or CP (creatinine phosphate). These high energy molecules cause the brain to think, the heart to pump blood, the muscles to lift weight and the sex organs to function on demand or spontaneously. We live because of the high energy molecules generated by sugar. Sugar provides quick energy. Energy is necessary for life and laughter, but if we eat more sugar than is required to live and laugh, sugar is stored as glycogen or fat.

Fat is composed of the same elements as sugar but in a much more complex form. Ninety-five percent (95%) of fat in the body is in the form of triglyceride, a molecule composed of glycerol and three fatty acids. These fatty acids are either saturated with hydrogen or unsaturated. Unsaturated fat is found in canola, olive and peanut oils and to some extent in safflower, sunflower, soybean and corn oils. Unsaturated fats are not as harmful to the body as saturated fats. Saturated fats are found in animal products including beef, lamb, pork and chicken. They are also present in egg yolk, cream, butter and cheese. In plants, saturated fats are present in coconut and palm oil, vegetable shortening and hydrogenated margarine. Food manufacturers use saturated fats in the making of cakes, cookies and pies.

There are some fats that are beneficial. The omega-3 fats found in cold water fish such as salmon, mackerel, sardines and tuna help protect against clots forming in arteries and thus protect against heart attacks and strokes.

In general, one should limit fat to less than 30% of daily energy needs. The saturated fats of egg yolks, cream, cheese, butter and vegetable oils should be studiously avoided. When cooking with oil, olive oil and canola are preferred. Remember, the healthiest fats are found in cold water fish.

Cholesterol is not truly a fat but since it behaves like one, it is commonly treated as a fat. Cholesterol is plentiful in egg yolk and meats, especially liver and kidney. It is also abundant in shellfish, particularly shrimp, and in dairy products such as cream, butter and whole milk. Cholesterol is not present in any vegetable.

Cholesterol not only is ingested from the animal sources cited, it is also manufactured in the body where it aids in building cell membranes and manufacturing hormones.

Cholesterol is carried in the blood stream by lipoproteins. High density lipoprotein cholesterol (HDL cholesterol) is "good" cholesterol, helping to protect against "hardening" of the arteries or atherosclerosis. Low density lipoprotein cholesterol (LDL cholesterol) is "bad" cholesterol, involved in causing atherosclerosis which is the prime cause of heart attack and strokes. Cholesterol in food should be avoided. The body manufactures enough for its own use. The avoidance of cholesterol means discipline and temperance in the consumption of large quantities of egg yolk, animal organ meats, shellfish and dairy products. The Tarahumara Indians of Mexico are primarily vegetarians and have an extremely low incidence of heart disease, cancer and stroke.

In summary, the avoidance of fat is the avoidance of heart disease, cancer and stroke. The total avoidance of fat is impossible, for vegetables contain oils which are fats and, in fact, a small amount of fat is necessary to carry into the body the beneficial fat soluble vitamins, A, D, E and K.

Fats kill, especially saturated fats, and cholesterol. Vegetarians live longer and better.

The body is built of protein. Protein, unlike carbohydrate and fat, is constructed not only of carbon, hydrogen and oxygen but also of nitrogen, sulfur, phosphorous and iron. Some protein is manufactured in the body, but most must be gained from foods. The foods most abundant in protein are meats, fish, poultry, eggs and dairy products. Cereals are 19% protein, vegetables are 7%, and beans, peas and nuts 5%. One could easily do without meat, fish and poultry and have a very sufficient supply of protein by having eggs, milk and vegetables (ovolactovegetarian diet).

To determine your daily requirement of protein multiply your normal healthy weight by 0.37.

The body continually undergoes breakdown and replacement. Hair falls out, the outer layer of skin continually sloughs off, the cells lining the gut die and are replaced, blood cells die in a certain number of days and are replaced from bone marrow, etc. Protein is necessary for this replacement. Additionally, some protein is used for energy, particularly when carbohydrate is low or when exercise is prolonged. Because protein can be used for energy, one must continue to provide oneself with protein when severely restricting carbohydrate to lose weight, otherwise the body destroys itself in search of energy.

Carbohydrate, fat and protein are our foods. Our lesson is to use them in a knowledgeable way, particularly when we wish to lose fat, but first we must examine some other nutrients.

Chapter IV

Vitamins, Antioxidants, Minerals, Water

Vitamins are micronutrients that aid in the energy actions of the body. The body can only manufacture vitamin D; all others are taken in with food.

Fat-soluble vitamins, A, D, E and K are stored in the fat cells of the body and used as needed. Vitamin A is found in green vegetables and milk products. It functions in the eyes and skin. Vitamin D is present in cod-liver oil, eggs and dairy products. It promotes the growth and maintenance of bone. Vitamin E is a constituent of seeds, green vegetables and margarine. It functions as an antioxidant to curtail free radicals that destroy body cells. Vitamin K is in green vegetables, cereals, fruits and meats. It is important in the blood clotting process. The water soluble vitamins, B-1, 2, 6, 12, niacin, pantothemic acid, folic acid, biotin and vitamin C are widely distributed in foods including meats, vegetables and dairy products. All of these vitamins act as coenzymes, which facilitate energy reactions. Vitamin C helps maintain bone and cartilage.

Since water soluble vitamins are dissolved in water, they are lost from the body in the urine and, therefore, must be taken in on a frequent basis.

Vitamins are necessary to the health of the body. When one is restricting food to lose fat, vitamins should be taken as a supplement.

There are 22 minerals in the body. They accrue in rivers, lakes, oceans, top soil and from ground below the earth surface, and we take them in through the food we eat and the water we drink. They function in three ways: they build the structure of the body, help to regulate the rhythm of the heart (the contraction of muscle) and send messages through the neural network, and are parts of regulators, enzymes.

Calcium and phosphorous are the most abundant minerals in the body. Together, calcium and phosphorous make up the majority of bones and teeth. Their loss or lack promotes osteoporosis and brittle bones. Milk products, sardines, canned salmon, kidney beans and dark leafy vegetables are good sources of calcium. In addition to its role in bones and teeth, phosphorous is a constituent of our old energy friends, adenosine triphosphate (ATP), adenosine diphosphate (ADP) and creatinine phosphate (CP). Phosphorous is found in milk products, meats and grains.

Magnesium helps store glucose as glycogen. It also helps break down glucose during energy reaction. It is found in whole grains and green leafy vegetables.

Iron is an essential part of the hemoglobin in red blood cells helping to carry oxygen into the body and carbon dioxide out. A deficiency of iron causes anemia. Iron is obtained from eggs, meats and green leafy vegetables.

Sodium, potassium and chlorine are termed electrolytes. They are charged particles distributed across cell membranes to keep an electrical balance, allowing the cell to live and work effectively. Our major source of sodium and chlorine is salt. Potassium is plentiful in fruits and fruit juices.

Chromium from fats, vegetable oils and meats helps bind insulin to cells in order to facilitate the transfer of glucose into cells. It is important when on a low carbohydrate diet to promote efficient use of what glucose is available.

Water constitutes 60-75% of the weight of the body. Its variation depends on the quantity of fat, for while water makes up 65-75% of muscle, only 25% is present in fat. Water is the means by which we live. It is a transport system for all things that come into the body and all that go out. It has tremendous heat stabilizing qualities, lubricates our joints and helps give us structure.

One should ingest at least 2.5 liters of water per day and more when performing physical activity. Water is generated from metabolism in the body, and ingested as pure water, water in food and water in all other liquids. It is lost from the skin, the lungs, urine and feces.

Water is a significant factor in helping the body lose fat, too much sodium, and retained water. Water suppresses appetite, making it easier to not eat too much. When the kidneys do not get enough water, they shift part of their load to the liver. Consequently, the liver slows down its fat burning process.

During a program to intentionally burn fat, at least 2.5 liters of water should be ingested daily.

Chapter V

Abnormal Body Composition

In Chapter II we saw the average body composition values for healthy persons of ages 20-22 years. These are values termed "reference man" (RM) and "reference woman" (RW). RM is 15% fat, 45% muscle, 15% bone and 25% other. RW is 25% fat, 38% muscle, 12% bone and 25% other.

Let's suppose RW weighs 125 pounds. Her body composition would look like this:

RW 125 lbs.		
	Pounds	% of Body Weight
Fat	31.25	25
Muscle	47.5	38
Bone	15	12
Other	31.25	25
Total	125	100

Let's suppose she becomes pregnant, gains significant weight and after delivery not only doesn't lose weight, but begins food binges and reaches 175 pounds within a year. Since the weight gain is mostly accumulated fat (muscle mass may actually increase with heavy weight gain due to having to carry more weight), she has gained fifty pounds of fat.

Her new (abnormal) body composition is:

RW 175 lbs.		
	Pounds	% of Body Weight
Fat	78.7	45
Muscle	50	28.5
Bone	15	8.5
Other	31.5	18
Total	175	100

RW is now an entirely different person. She must not only carry her new child around but also fifty extra pounds of fat. The extra weight is analogous to wearing a backpack with 50 pounds of bricks that must be worn in bed, in the bathroom, while shopping, while socializing, and at church. She is constantly tired, doesn't have enough energy for all her work, doesn't like her looks, gets less attention from her husband and has had to acquire a completely new wardrobe. She is emotionally drained, feels self-conscious and is frustrated by the inability to curb her appetite. Her altered body composition has made her ill. She is at risk for diabetes, hypertension, cancer, heart disease, a stroke or other malady, if she can not regain her former health.

Chapter VI

Causes of Being Overweight

A. Genetic

We are made of the stuff of our parents. My parents were of small to moderate frame. My mother was judicious in her eating and lived to 99 years. My father's sole joy in life was food and he was overweight. He lived until 74, his death set in motion by an oversight on the part of his physician. One of my patient's mothers was of moderate frame and she was adamant regarding proper nutrition. She was never overweight. Her husband was large and rotund. My patient and her brother struggle with weight. Many of my other patients tell exactly the same story.

Many of my overweight patients not only tell the story of their overweight parents but they also relate the history of diabetes, cancer, stroke, Alzheimer's and other problems frequently related to obesity.

Despite the strong influence of genetic factors associated with obesity, there is no force stronger than determination in losing weight and maintaining that loss.

B. Situational

When I first interview a person who has come to me to learn to lose and control weight, I patiently coax them into telling me about their guess as to why they have gained too much weight. Many tell the same tale. They gradually have adapted to the situation of their lives. Most have a spouse who loves and requires an abundance of food, especially food that is tasteful, sweet and fat. Their children demand grits, waffles, butter, syrup, pancakes, bacon, sausage, whole milk and cheese. Their grandchildren come to visit for a week or long weekends. Their habit is Coke, Pepsi, Gingerale, doughnuts, cookies, ice cream. When the family is away, the neighbors come for the card party with the hors d' oeuvres and wine. When the neighbors are gone, the invitation lays waiting on the kitchen counter to the cocktail party tomorrow night with the wine, cheese, shrimp, crab, sandwiches and chips.

Most of my patients tell me about the temptation of food. They simply ask how to control it.

C. Stress

Of all the factors related to being overweight, the most severe is stress. Stress is that part of life which by its influence causes us discomfort. It may be anything, the tone of voice of our spouse, the pressure of our job, the need to repair part of the house, the failing health of parents, impending divorce, illness, death in the family. Whatever the stress, the most frequent tendency is to run. Running is the natural human reflex; confrontation is far more difficult. Running takes many forms but the most frequent is to find some immediate way of becoming satisfied and that most frequent way is to eat something, something good, like sweets or fat.

Stress is that which makes us uncomfortable, food makes us comfortable, and so the battle wages, constantly. Only when we recognize that which is stressful can we build a wall between stress and us.

D. Job

A few jobs are by chance healthy. Soldiers, sailors, lumberjacks and farmers all have jobs which by their nature are too demanding and too physically strenuous to allow time and food to be overly influential. Most of us are not soldiers, sailors and the like. Doctors and lawyers are sedentary; preachers have a bite at every household. Teachers eat a good breakfast, have an unhealthy lunch and fix a big dinner at night. Nurses snack. Firemen sit around. Policemen hustle from one fast food joint to another. Many businessmen lunch, a lot.

A job can be healthy or not. Again, the trick is to recognize the influence on our eating habits and to design our healthy life patterns around our job rather than letting the job subtly guide us into being overweight.

E. Social

Among my many delightful patients, some are more intense than others. They are persons who quickly relate to others, enjoy conversation, gain pleasure from others and easily fit the category of being "people persons." Moreover, those people persons who are fortunate to have sufficient wealth to not have to work design their lives to constantly party. All parties are peripherally constructed around a table or tables of food. The food itself is the best that the hostess could find. The fruit is piled high, the bread has been shorn of its crust and the tiny sausages have been wrapped in bacon. My most social patients wonder why they have gained weight.

F. Knowledge

No one ever teaches us what to eat. My delightful childhood had at its center the breakfast, lunch and dinner table. With doting parents, four siblings, and a full-time cook, our meals were among my most pleasant memories of family. Sunday dinner (lunch) after church was impressive. Fat fried chicken, butter beans, rice, biscuits, iced tea with several spoonfuls of sugar preceded dessert.

Never during my many years of formal education did any teacher ever stress the need to carefully tailor foods for health.

The cause of being overweight is too much food. Even today, with recognition that the major debilitating and death providers are food, there are few single resources to guide our paths to correct food programs.

Knowledge of foods, their caloric content, their fat, saturated fat, carbohydrate, protein content, vitamin and mineral content is mandatory for the ability to live a healthy and reasonably long life.

G. Contact

Few people can live without social contact and be healthy doing so. Most need contact and all overweight persons need knowledgeable contact. Most weight management programs fail and all weight management programs fail without a physician specialist in weight management. The most successful weight management centers have an endocrinologist at the command post and other physicians who have come to learn weight management as patient contacts. Contact does not have to be lengthy but does need to be frequent, generally every two weeks. Physician contact, even by telephone, teaches the patient what foods are good and bad for him or her as an individual. Contact teaches which situational, environmental, social or other influence is providing impediment or success to that person's program.

Contact teaches motivation and it is the primary factor that provides proper weight maintenance.

H. Hormonal

While many of the body's hormones may be operative in the cause or effect of being overweight or obese, two are of important and immediate association.

Thyroxine is manufactured by the thyroid gland in the neck. The thyroid gland is under the influence of the pituitary gland in the brain. The pituitary gland is in turn controlled by the amount of thyroxine liberated by the thyroid gland. Thus, there is a balance, the pituitary stimulating the thyroid and the thyroid controlling the stimulation by the pituitary. All is well when there is a balance between these two glands. The thyroxine liberated by the thyroid gland influences the rate at which the body works. When there is too much thyroxine the body revs up, the heart beats faster, there is generalized nervousness, the body heats up, causing heat intolerance, and the person is agitated. When there is not enough thyroxine, metabolism slows down. Now there is sluggishness, depression and cold intolerance. Hypothyroidism, as this latter condition is called, is far more prevalent than is generally regarded. Roughly twenty percent (one in five) overweight adult women have hypothyroidism. Many of these women have normal blood values for thyroxine and thyroid stimulating hormone but have diminished receptor function where thyroxine acts. Diminished receptor function is not measured in conventional blood analyses. Moreover, when an overweight woman having diminished thyroid function severely restricts her diet, the thyroid condition worsens, her metabolism slows down and it becomes difficult or impossible for her to continue to lose weight. At this point, the contact physician must recognize her symptoms and administer thyroid hormone.

A second major hormonal situation associated with fat accumulation is diagnosed with blood analysis of insulin. Insulin is a powerful hormone manufactured by the beta cells of the pancreas. One of insulin's major functions is to facilitate the entrance of glucose into cells. When one ingests a high carbohydrate meal, the pancreas liberates insulin in appropriate amounts to sweep the glucose into cells for use in providing energy or to store it as glycogen or fat. When a diet is chronically high in carbohydrate, insulin remains high in the blood stream, becoming less and less effective in handling glucose. This imbalance can lead eventually to diabetes. Another effect of high insulin values is that it depresses glucagon, a hormone that promotes the liberation of fat from storage. If meals contain moderate carbohydrate, insulin is not chronically elevated and glucagon can be effective in diminishing fat storage.

Most physicians do not test for insulin and, therefore, miss its important role in weight management and the prevention of diabetes.

I. Age

There aren't many fat old people. Fat kills.

The aging process is a long and complicated function. It is discernible in the average population at about thirty years, slowly but steadily is seen in all organ systems until about age seventy and then proceeds more rapidly until death. The best current theory of the cause of aging is the free radical theory. Free radicals are oxygen containing molecules that have an extra electron. They donate this extra electron to membranes and life sustaining molecules like DNA (deoxyribonucleic acid). The membrane or DNA is damaged by the electron causing it to malfunction (age). Free radicals are a natural occurrence in the body's energy reactions but are held in check by antioxidants which "steal" the extra electron before it can do damage. Free radicals are also caused by exercise, sunlight, radiation and smoking. One cigarette can generate thousands of free radicals. Smoking is associated with heart disease, lung cancer, and premature aging. Research in thousands of experiments during the past fifty years has shown the protective effect of antioxidants in the aging process and specifically in the prevention of conditions such as heart disease, cancer, stroke and premature aging. Antioxidants are attained from foods. Some foods, rich in vitamins (C & E are antioxidants) and antioxidants are beans, blueberries, broccoli, oats, pumpkin, wild salmon, green tea, walnuts and yogurt.

J. Sex

Eighty-five to ninety percent of the patients in our weight management center are women. Most of them first became overweight during their first pregnancy and have never been strict enough to return to their prenatal body composition. As we have seen there are many pressures to make it difficult to return to previous normal body composition: spouses, children, jobs, stress, social, etc. If one adds to this the prevalence of subclinical thyroiditis that slows down metabolism, and the enormous quantity of food available, then being overweight is easy. Once the weight is obvious, discomforting, and associated with disease states, women want the advice of a physician experienced in weight management. Prime among their motivation, are looks, wardrobe and social acceptance.

Men determined to lose weight are generally advised to do so for health reasons. Heart disease, cancer and stroke, the major killers are all associated with obesity. Once the male decides to lose weight, he generally does so with speed and effectiveness.

When either sex loses significant weight, both state an increase in energy, self satisfaction and a determination to keep from gaining again.

Chapter VII

Complications

A. Diabetes Mellitus

Diabetes mellitus is one of the most frequent complications of obesity. The person typical of impending diabetes frequently has a high fasting blood sugar, high triglycerides (fat in the blood), high total cholesterol, high low-density lipoprotein cholesterol, and a high fasting blood insulin level. The higher the insulin (result of having eaten too much carbohydrate), the greater the blood sugar level (insulin more ineffective in keeping blood sugar level constant). Diabetes is not a sudden event. Damage to elevated sugar levels may occur years before the doctor says "diabetes." When sugar levels are chronically high, nerves and arteries are damaged, producing diabetes as a painful debilitating condition.

B. Hypertension

High blood pressure is caused by arterial damage and by vasoconstriction (spasm of arteries). Stress and being overweight are the most frequent conditions associated with hypertension. When blood vessels are damaged to the extent that the heart must pump harder, the heart itself will begin to suffer and heart failure may be the eventual result. When blood pressure is elevated and high low-density lipoprotein cholesterol presents, atherosclerosis (hardening of the arteries) is accelerated (frequently in the arteries of the heart). If clots form on one of the diseased arteries, a heart attack or stroke may occur.

The best medicine to prevent hypertension is weight control.

C. Heart Attack

A heart attack results from the closure of one or more of the coronary arteries. The heart is a muscular pump. It pumps five liters of blood per minute, less when resting, more when doing physical activity. As with all the muscles in the body, it is fed food, water and oxygen constantly. The coronary arteries begin in the aorta (the major artery leaving the heart), deliver their food, water and oxygen, and then empty into veins leaving the heart. The heart can tolerate a temporary change in food and water but can not tolerate any cessation of its oxygen supply. With hypertension and high cholesterol, damage occurs to the coronary arteries as it does to other arteries in the body. This damage is gradual, occurring just below the interior surface of the artery causing it to bulge inward. These hard bulges are called plaques. Eventually, plaque may close the entire artery in a gradual manner causing severe chest pain (angina pectoris) or it may rupture suddenly, causing abrupt chest pain or death. Frequently these plaques are associated with blood clots, which also can occlude the coronary artery and cause heart attacks.

The prevention of heart attack is the prevention of hardening of the arteries (atherosclerosis). Since atherosclerosis is caused by too much fat in the blood (triglycerides and low density lipoprotein cholesterol) then heart attacks can be prevented by reducing fat consumption, and consuming only the amount of fat and carbohydrate necessary to maintain the body and to do one's daily work.

D. Stroke

The most prevalent cause of stroke is similar to atherosclerosis in the coronary arteries of the heart. The muscles of the heart are fed by these coronary arteries. Strokes are caused by atherosclerosis of the carotid arteries that originate in the chest and carry blood containing oxygen and glucose to the brain. These arteries are particularly prone to atherosclerosis in their mid portions in the neck. The complication is the same. The atherosclerotic plaque bulges into the interior of the artery until it occludes the artery and cuts off blood supply to the brain. Sometime the plaque ruptures before it occludes the major artery and parts of it are carried into the smaller arteries of the brain causing more specific symptoms such as minor strokes or specific loss of function of a body part. Again, blood clots play a dangerous role in causing strokes.

The prevention of strokes is the same as the prevention of heart attacks: the prevention of atherosclerosis. The prevention of atherosclerosis is to eat only what is needed for body maintenance and the doing of work.

E. Cancer

The causes of cancer are myriad. Cancer is the loss of control of the normal replacement of body cells. Cancers are runaway engines. The abnormal accelerated growth of abnormal cells causes tumors (cancers) that destroy the normal function of body organs.

Despite the multiple influences, which may cause this lack of control and accelerate abnormal growth, being overweight or obese is the most frequent associated condition with cancer (exceptions are the more specific causes such as smoking with lung cancer).

The healthiest people on this planet, and those with the lowest rate of cancer, are those who maintain a normal body composition by eating only that which best maintains the body and provides energy for doing work.

F. Liver Damage

The liver is said to be the most important organ in the body, doing some of the body's most complicated chemical work. My professor of biochemistry liked to say that the legs were for the purpose of transporting the liver around, the gut was to bring food to the liver, the lungs and heart were to breathe and pump blood for the liver, the brain was to instruct what to eat for the liver and the sex organs were for the purpose of generating more livers.

The three most prevalent conditions that damage the liver are infection (hepatitis), alcoholism (cirrhosis) and fat (fatty liver). All cause dysfunction of the liver and possible death. The most dramatic sign of severe liver damage is jaundice. Bile made by the liver for digestion purposes, backs up in the dysfunctional liver and causes a yellow-green coloration of the skin. Of the three causes, fatty liver is the subtlest, frequently occurring over many years and often associated with excessive alcohol intake. The liver manufactures a large number of important enzymes and blood analysis of these enzymes may lead to early diagnosis of fatty liver.

The prevention of hepatitis is care of vaccinations for travel in third world countries, abstinence of continued drug use and appropriate use of antibiotics when needed. The prevention of cirrhosis is the abstinence or moderation of the use of alcohol. The prevention of fatty liver is to avoid fat and excessive carbohydrates.

G. Hypercholesterolemia

Cholesterol is a substance that looks, feels, and behaves like a fat.

Cholesterol is manufactured in the body mainly to aid in forming hormones, the building of cell membranes and the synthesis of vitamin D. Cholesterol is not only manufactured in our bodies but also is found in other animal tissues. The richest source of cholesterol is egg yolk. Cholesterol is also concentrated in red meats, liver, shell fish and dairy products.

There are three major types of cholesterol in the blood stream that can be analyzed and give an indication of the quantity of cholesterol in the body. High density lipoprotein cholesterol (HDL-C) is called "good" cholesterol because it is a molecule that helps transport cholesterol out of the body where it can do no harm. The quantity of HDL-C is influenced by genetic factors, balanced diet and exercise. "Bad" cholesterol occurs most frequently in two forms, low density lipoprotein cholesterol (LDL-C) and very low density lipoprotein cholesterol (VLDL-C). Bad cholesterol is the culprit in causing atherosclerosis. It deposits cholesterol fractions beneath the cells lining arteries, which causes a type of "inflammatory" reaction. This reaction is the basis of forming an atherosclerotic plaque that may eventually cause heart attack or stroke.

The quantity of cholesterol in the blood should not exceed 200 milligrams, and a high proportion of this should be "good" cholesterol.

The control of cholesterol is control of eating animal products such as egg yolk, red meat, shellfish and dairy products.

H. Hyperinsulinemia

Insulin is one of the most important hormones in the body. Its prime function is to regulate the entrance of glucose into body cells. When a meal high in carbohydrate, especially when composed of simple sugars, is ingested, blood levels of glucose rise rapidly. When these increasing levels of glucose are noted by the pancreas, its beta cells pour out their supply of insulin. The insulin then travels with the glucose to the cells of the body and there facilitates the entrance of glucose into the cell's interior. In the interior of the cell, it is used for energy and if there is more than enough, it is stored as glycogen. When there is enough glycogen, it is stored as fat.

When the blood glucose level falls by virtue of its use or storage, the pancreas notes the lower level and shuts off the supply of insulin.

When the beta cells of the pancreas are destroyed by viruses, particularly in childhood and youth, the manufacture of insulin is severely curtailed. Without insulin the youth becomes severely ill, for his cells can no longer work without the energy from glucose. Glucose levels rise, glucose is lost in the urine, carrying with it large quantities of body water. During this phase, large quantities of fat are burned, causing acidosis and severe debilitation. The condition is now called Type I or juvenile diabetes mellitus and must be treated with insulin injections.

Adult diabetes results from progressive insult to the pancreas by too much food and alcohol. Damage to the pancreas is much slower and less severe than in the near total loss of beta cells in the juvenile. The subtler onset of Type II or maturity-onset diabetes makes it more difficult to see it coming. The single best yard stick for predicting the onset of adult diabetes in the level of insulin in the blood after a 12-18 hour lack of food. After a fast, the blood insulin should drop to below 6.0. When it does not, it is indicative of a chronic high carbohydrate diet overworking the pancreas, causing insulin resistance at the cellular level and leaving a chronically elevated level of insulin, hyperinsulinemia. The only problem with this simple, highly accurate predictive tool is that most physicians do not use it, not fully understanding its implications. The other less specific indicator of hyperinsulinemia is weight. The more one weighs over a longer period of time, the more likely the presence of hyperinsulinemia and the more possible the eventual onset of adult diabetes.

Prevention of hyperinsulinemia is the prevention of loading the body with unnecessary carbohydrates.

Chapter VIII

Weight Management Plan

Most weight management plans (food diets) do not work. They do not work because they are not knowledge based, are not directed by medical, physiological and psychology professionals or are originally misconceived. Original misconception includes the Atkins diet that recommends low carbohydrate but normal levels of fat. If you eat fat beyond need, you are going to deposit fat, look fat, feel fat and be fat. The Zone Diet touts a zone. There is no zone, there is only reality. Jenny Craig and Weight Watchers do not work because of the lack of professional advisors.

A Weight Management plan that does work is this one. It is composed of ten basic elements:

A. Knowledge
B. Motivation
C. Determination
D. Contact
E. Goals
F. Food substitution
G. Appetite suppression
H. Pharmaceuticals
I. Nutriceuticals
J. Physical activity

A. Knowledge
You have already gained a significant amount of knowledge. You have learned that 70% of American adults are either overweight or obese. You have learned:

- Normal body composition and how to calculate your Body Mass Index

- That all food can be classed as carbohydrate, fat or protein and that a good weight management plan to low weight should be one of curtailing carbohydrates and fat and maintaining a normal amount of protein
- The nature and importance of vitamins, antioxidants, minerals and water
- Abnormal body composition and its consequences
- The most frequent causes of becoming overweight or obese
- The serious complications of obesity

The preceding is a greater amount of knowledge than most people have and more than many physicians and other "advisors" practice. There is no end to emerging knowledge concerning this subject because of emerging interest in obesity and its being the single most important medical condition today. Additionally, we have sought not to drown those interested in this subject but to gently float them on a raft amid a sea of misconceptions. My colleagues and I offer simple, true, easily understood knowledge. We do so continuously by maintaining contact on a frequent basis with anyone undertaking our program.

B. Motivation

Motivation is not a psychological drama. It begins slowly, imperceptibly. It may begin when the belt is loosened, the shirt collar chokes or the dress won't fit. It is there at a glance in the mirror, when your feet hurt, when you puff up the stairs. It comes slamming home when the doctor says "You should lose some weight." Motivation is always there, mostly unrecognized, but always disturbing. It is like a pot of water on the stove, warm, heating, steaming, sizzling and finally coming to an explosive boil. That is when motivation faces you squarely and says "I'm gonna lose weight. I'm going to have to see an expert, and want a personal trainer."

C. Determination

There is an old saying "Persistence and perseverance made a Bishop of his Reverence." You can be a Bishop if you are determined. Determination is within the hands of most. It is most frequently seen in intelligent persons who have succeeded because they had determination, and it is frequently manifest in those who have had to confront difficult situations whether they succeeded or not. One of the most determined persons I have ever known is one of my sons. When he was only a baby (approximately one year old), he preferred to stay up when we watched TV. We preferred to put him in bed at a relatively early hour. His response was to cry. Our eventual response was "Well, let him cry for a while, he will tire and go to sleep like all babies and a little crying is not going to hurt him." When a half hour passed we looked at each other. At an hour he was watching TV with us. It never hurt him. Later, I watched, with pain, his determination to ride his new bicycle in our back yard. After he fell countless times and I was a broken man, he rode.

Entering a new program with new trainees in the current era of myth and misinformation can be a daunting experience. Success will much depend on determination, and determination is not easily consistent. One has to begin with a large amount and mete it out constantly along the way. You, too, can become a Bishop.

D. Contact

Contact is singularly important. Your contact must be a medically trained Personal Trainer. Your "Personal Trainer" may be derived in multiple ways, but must be frequently or constantly available. The plan will not work without this contact. The contact, however expressed, must have a constant, easily remembered wealth of knowledge derived from medical, physiological and psychological training.

Beyond the medical training, the base for your contact must be entirely devoted to you in the focused arena of weight management. Even more importantly, your contact must have had significant training and experience in the everyday reality of weight management practice.

Your contact is your Personal Trainer, preferably being available on a daily basis, ready to provide information, encourage and guide you to a healthy lifestyle you can maintain for the rest of your healthy, happy life.

E. Goals

My wife has a Global Positioning System (GPS) in her car. It is of significant advantage, for she once asked me what a compass does. She once left Asheville, NC, with our daughter to come back to Charleston, SC, and had to turn around in Tennessee. She now dials in her destination in the GPS and it not only displays an easy to follow multicolored map but it talks to her all the way. Interestingly, she talks back. My daughter told me these things. I don't mention them.

Once motivation prompts and determination becomes ironclad, a realistic goal should be approached, not set. This goal should be shared with the Personal Trainer, even if it has been predetermined. It is well not to set as a goal a specific weight, especially if that weight is one of youth or early maturity. The body inevitably changes after age thirty. The rest of our life should be composed of making those changes occur as slowly as possible. Having babies creates changes. Being of age to play two sets of tennis, rather than four, creates changes. Having enough money to buy food, rather than swipe it off the patients' trays, creates changes. Setting a specific weight may create unneeded frustration when the last ten pounds appear impossible. A better set of goals are more realistic parameters, such as a combination of significant weight loss, more energy, satisfaction with personal appearance, a better wardrobe and a keen sense of satisfaction. Our patients who set realistic goals and faithfully follow our program have a 100% success rate. Success breeds good long-term maintenance. Our patients are happy, even joyous, at their success in having set realistic goals and attaining them. My wife is always happy when she reaches her destination. She has her personal trainer GPS, sets proper goals, and is always successful.

F. Food substitution

My youngest son became seriously ill at seven years of age. My wife diagnosed the illness as diabetes before her doctor husband did. She demanded immediate attention from one of my specialist colleagues who regarded her as much of a drill sergeant as I did. My son and my wife were hospitalized on a pediatric diabetes ward where they learned carbohydrate substitution among other matters of proper diabetes management. I went down to Market Street where shops sold junk to tourists and bought him a sword. He was delighted and kept it in his bed clearly visible to the terror stricken nurses who came to give him shots.

This program is founded on scientifically formulated substitutions for meals ordinarily containing too many carbohydrates. While demanding a low fat regimen, its prime power is diminishing carbohydrates to the point where the body burns its stored carbohydrates and fats. This is not easy. One pound of fat contains 3,500 calories (actually kilocalories, written as a big C when expressed as Calories. The word will be used with a little c by current convention). To lose one pound of fat, the body must be denied 3,500 calories. The loss of six pounds of fat over a two week period represents denying the body 21,000 calories.

To attain this kind of result (which represents a good average), one must strike fat from his food intake by selecting meats and dairy products without appreciable fats (fish, wild game, trimmed pork, poultry without skin, egg without yolk, and skim milk).

The key, however, which has been lost on the American public, is the denial of carbohydrate. Fat is bad in the American diet, carbohydrate is the villain. Fully 80% of everything in a modern American grocery store is carbohydrate.

Our method of proving weight loss is substitution for carbohydrate. The substitutes are easily prepared, scientifically researched packets containing protein, minerals and a rich array of vitamins and antioxidants. One packet contains 100 calories, significant protein (30% of daily requirement) and a tiny amount of fat (3% of usual daily intake). The vitamins and minerals are sufficient and are complemented by additional vitamins and minerals in other forms.

The packet is a powder and comes in numerous forms and flavors. Chocolate is a favorite flavor with strawberry and cappuccino running close seconds. Cheese cake, mocha and chocolate mint are also available. These packets contain powdered nutrients which are easily soluble in water, ice or skim milk in an electric blender. Blended in this way, they are often referred to as "shakes."

Several of our programs are constructed around the substitution of shakes for meals. The simplest and most effective program is "Total" substitution. In the "Total" program there is complete substitution of shakes for all food. A shake is substituted for breakfast, lunch and dinner with a shake at mid-afternoon and another prior to bed. A person on the Total Program is thus restricted to 500 calories per day instead of his usual 2000 or 2500 calories. Carbohydrate storage is rapidly depleted and fat begins to burn like a forest fire. On such a determined program, it is not uncommon to lose 10-12 pounds per two week period. Many go four to six weeks on the Total, an occasional person commits to 10-12 weeks.

More frequently, a person jump-starts with 1-2 weeks on Total and then switches to "Moderate." The Moderate program has two forms, "Moderate 2 + 2" and "Moderate 3 + 1. Moderate 2 + 2 consists of having a shake substitution for breakfast, lunch of salad with "lite" salad dressing, a shake at mid-afternoon and dinner consisting of low carbohydrate vegetables and a small amount of low fat meat such as fish, skinless chicken or turkey, fat trimmed pork or wild game such as venison. The Moderate 2 + 2 is thus a program of 2 shakes and 2 meals. The Moderate 3 + 1 varies only by selecting 3 shakes and 1 meal. The choice between these two programs generally depends on lifestyle and job requirements. Both are equally effective.

Meal substitution is not confined to the shakes mentioned above. Also available are a variety of similarly prepared soups, juices, hot drinks and snack bars to fit erratic schedules, travel plans and unpredictable job requirements.

The entire food substitution concept is simply an effective means of changing food habits which have led to being overweight or obese to a disciplined and necessary self-inspection of what foods are really composed of and which are suitable for whom.

It is extremely effective and extraordinarily simple. When one commits to 500-1000 calories instead of 2000-3000 calories, weight is lost, 100% of the time. The greatest asset, however, is knowledge, the inevitable learning of what all foods are composed of and which specific foods hold hidden qualities. When a person is denied fruit on these programs, he naturally questions why and learns of enormous quantities of glucose and fructose in fruit. He learns that white foods, bread, pasta, potatoes, rice and cereals are laden with carbohydrates. He learns that meats carefully selected for their naturally low fat (venison) or those shorn of fat (skinless poultry) are quite permissible and contain necessary protein. He also learns that when he has reached his goals set early in the program that he can return to food more carefully selected than in his former life without detriment to himself.

Food substitution is a simple and effective means to lose weight and generates a learning process not taught anywhere in his former life, not by his mother, not by any school, not by society and not by fad diets.

The key to this excellent learning process is constant contact with the Personal Trainer. The trainer will continually provide motivation, reinforce determination, exude encouragement, congratulate success and build knowledge. The Personal Trainer can achieve these successes because of medical, scientific, psychology background, experience in the weight management field and an orderly, well organized knowledge base.

G. Appetite Suppressants

An appetite suppressant is a medication which keeps one from feeling hungry. By itself, it does not cause weight loss, for the appetite (hunger) always returns, prompting us to eat. Hunger is composed of two elements, one central, in the brain which says "eat", and which is stimulated by the level of glucose in the blood, the quantity of insulin and other hormones and the state of the intestinal distention and content.

Fat is a natural appetite suppressant. Eskimos, gorging on fat, are not hungry. Carbohydrates, especially, simple sugars, provoke an immediate and high insulin response from the pancreas, which has a rapid effect on the hypothalamus in the brain and causes a sensation of immediate hunger. A distended stomach or a surgically improvised small one provides satiety; a large, undistended stomach signals hunger from the hypothalamus via the vagal nerve.

Appetite is a complex brain-engineered entity which says either "eat" or nothing.

Appetite suppressants are an appropriate and important part of a weight management program. There are many chemical appetite suppressants, some natural, some yet to be found or perfected, some tried and taken away by the Federal Drug Administration by virtue of suggestion but yet unproven assertions.

Phentermine hydrochloride in 37.5 mgm tablets, used once per day or broken to use half a tablet in the morning and half at noon is the best appetite suppressant on the market. It has been extensively used, and used reasonably, it is free of serious side effects.

Phentermine exerts its effect centrally, in the brain, freeing norepinephrine from nerve endings. It is thus a stimulant, can interfere with sleep, cause agitation and nervousness and exacerbate higher blood pressure in hypertensive patients. Used rationally, after good advice, it can substantially ameliorate the pangs of hunger.

An appetite suppressant does not cause weight loss; it simply makes the disciplined process of voluntary food control, tolerable.

H. Pharmaceuticals

Fortunately, there are not many drugs to consider as appropriate or necessary in the management of weight. More importantly, it is crucial to consider the advantage that proper weight management provides in the lack of necessity to take a myriad of drugs. Frequently the person considered a Type II diabetic is receiving 4-5 medications to control his diabetes. Weight loss obviates all of them. When beginning this weight loss program, we would cut all of their diabetes medication in half and later remove most, if not all. The same is true of antidepressant medications. Persons losing significant weight feel better about themselves, have more confidence, less depression and function better. Weight loss also has an immediate and significant effect on hypertension. "Blood pressure medicines" are soon thrown away as unnecessary. Medicines designed to control hypercholesterolemia are unnecessary after one learns to avoid cholesterol laden meats and becomes more focused upon healthy vegetables and non-meat proteins (beans, eggs, and dairy products). The latter is termed an ovo-(egg) lacto-(milk) vegetarian diet.

There are, however, a few medications to consider when embarking upon a serious weight management program amidst a sea of complicating circumstances. If, upon starting a weight loss program, blood glucose is found to be relatively high and blood insulin to be significantly high in the fasting state (>12 mgm), glucophage (Metformin) 500 mgm per day is indicated. Glucophage acts by interfering with gluconeogenesis (formation of new sugar from protein) in the liver, thus sparing the insulin its overworked control of glucose until the body normalizes. Glucophage can be used in higher doses but occasionally provides irritable gastrointestinal symptoms and has to be discontinued. Prolonged carbohydrate restriction will eventually solve the hyperinsulinemia without the necessity of glucophage.

A much more frequently needed medication is thyroxine. Let's review, for a moment, the role of the thyroid gland in obesity. The thyroid gland in the neck, upon stimulation by the pituitary gland in the brain, produces levothyroxine (T4). T4 is an inactive hormone but is converted to T3 by a process called deiodination (loss of iodine). T3 stimulates the metabolic process, causing the engine to run faster. An over amount of T3 causes restlessness, lack of sleep, apprehension, fast pulse rate, sweating, heat intolerance, <u>weight loss</u>. When there is not enough T3, or when the receptors at the organ sites where it affects its results, become insensitive to its effects (T3 resistance), the person involved feels depressed, sleepy, unenergetic, has a slow pulse rate, has cold intolerance and gains weight.

It is estimated that twenty percent (20%) of adult American women have encountered viruses which have caused an inflammatory condition of their thyroid glands known as Hashimoto's thyroiditis. These women are thyroid hormone deficient and are prone to gain weight despite trying to live a reasonable work and food lifestyle.

Not only is a hypothyroid (low thyroid hormone output) condition likely to be present in a large group of overweight women, but the very process of trying to correct their overweight condition exacerbates a diminution of thyroid hormone output. When the food input of a person trying to lose weight is severely restricted, the thyroid gland simply quits putting out the usual thyroid hormone as a response. It is like being thrown in jail. The body says "Oh, lord, they've thrown us in jail and they are not feeding us, let's go sit down in the corner and not move." Metabolism decreases. The person who was doing well losing weight suddenly hits a plateau and can't lose any more despite a severe dietary restriction. The general medical public denies this circumstance citing that the blood values for the thyroid hormone components are within "the normal range." The general medical public is looking at laboratory values rather than the patient and her circumstances. Under these circumstances it is imperative to give the patient assistance with levothyroxine (T4) or thyroid extract (T3), or both. Upon giving sufficient external hormone support, the patient is quickly relieved symptomatically, and continues her weight loss progress. Occasionally, the justified administration of thyroid hormone, during a dieting program, is a dramatic relief. More often, it is a gradual but gratifying process and can be well monitored by simply providing constant patient contact with the Personal Trainer.

I.   Nutriceuticals

A properly founded nutritional program assures that food (carbohydrate, fat, protein) is sufficient and that vitamins, antioxidants, minerals and water are sufficient.

A seriously restricted food program (low fat, low carbohydrate, normal protein) must do the same. One can seriously restrict carbohydrate and the body will burn fat for energy, manufacture new carbohydrate from protein (must supply adequate protein) and not suffer in the process. The only additional consideration is to provide vitamins, minerals, anti-oxidants and water in amounts sufficient to maintain optimal health. From this consideration the Personal Trainer advises:

1. Fiber in the form of oat bran, one 850 mg capsule per day.
2. Potassium one 600 mg capsule per day to supplement the restriction of fruit and fruit juices.
3. Calcium, one 500 mg capsule to supplement the restriction of dairy products including cheese.
4. Multivitamins, including antioxidants C and E.
5. Chromium, one capsule 200mcg to aid insulin in the facilitated diffusion of glucose into body cells.
6. Water, at least two liters per day, and the more, the better.

J. Physical Activity

There is a common misconception that the way to lose weight is by exercise. One only need look at a variety of very good athletes to see the variation of truth in this common misconception. Begin with the sumo wrestler and end with the marathoner and you will view a rainbow of associations to exercise and fat.

For those not occupied with running, racing 26 miles, or being thrown out of the ring by another fat person, the path to trimness is to eat only what we need, not that exercise is bad. Exercise is good, good for our bones, good for body muscles, good for the special muscle, the heart, and good for the mind. The mind benefits especially from exercise. When I used to run habitually, I floated. I enjoyed the air, the sun, even a light rain. As my run progressed, my endorphins kicked in and I could not only <u>not</u> feel the run but I could feel a special elation. I was even happier after the run. It had been a good run and I was satisfied. I remained trim, my muscles were right and I bounced as I walked. Exercise is good, but when one seeks to lose excess weight, care must be taken.

The first week of a serious curtailment of food depletes the sugar stored as glycogen. The average person stores 400-500 grams of carbohydrate. Since each gram is capable of giving 4 calories of energy or 1600-2000 calories total, all of the stored carbohydrate could be depleted in an intense 2 hour exercise period. In high performance athletes, this depletion is called "bonking" or "hitting the wall."

When one confines his intake of energy to 500 calories as on the Total program, glycogen is rapidly depleted. With less energy, fatigue begins during exercise, especially while on a low carbohydrate diet, onsets earlier and is more severe than usual. Even the psyche plays differently during the early phase of a low carbohydrate diet. Persons on a low carbohydrate diet are often more irritable during the first week of the diet. If one is taught to expect this possibility and is reminded of it by the Personal Trainer, mood swings can be controlled. In summary, when one doesn't put as much gas in the tank, the engine won't run as long.

As the body adapts to the new food program, exercise becomes more permissible. Walking is a particularly good exercise while on a carbohydrate restricted diet. Walking at 3 miles per hour causes a 160 pound person to expend 4.5 calories per minute or only 135 total calories in 30 minutes. The effect is negligible (the number of calories in an apple) but provides a satisfying effect.

Running at a mild rate for one mile and walking one mile uses essentially the same amount of energy except for the fact that running is slightly less efficient so burns a few more calories. The prime difference is the time used.

Weight training exercise (resistance exercise) is again of little effect on the capacity to lose fat but produces an interesting effect. Weight training produces more muscle, more muscle means more capability to burn carbohydrates and fat, so weight training is beneficial in the long run although not effective in taking fat away in the early phases of a weight management program. An interesting aspect of weight training while dieting is that if one builds muscle at the same rate as he loses fat, his weight won't change.

Exercise is good, but combining it with a low carbohydrate, low fat food intake is the path to better body composition.

Chapter IX

Integration

We have seen that the Personal Trainer Program consists of:

1. Knowledge
2. Motivation
3. Determination
4. Contact
5. Goals
6. Food substitution
7. Appetite suppressants
8. Pharmaceuticals
9. Neutriceuticals
10. Physical activity

In this last chapter we shall integrate the above into a real life program which has been shown to have a 100% success rate in those who use it as it is designed.

The process begins when a person signs in at our clinic. A thorough medical history is taken including all current medical conditions and medications. Particularly important is family history which gives clues as to the possibilities of heart disease, stroke, cancer, thyroid dysfunction, diabetes, etc. Recent illness may make it inadvisable to begin the program until stability is certain. Current medications need to be carefully studied and it has been found that many are totally unnecessary.

In addition to the medical history, a lengthy personal history is obtained. It reveals the person's job, hobbies, recreation, usual physical activity, exercise patterns, employment and social preferences. Subtly, it probes for personality traits such as introversion versus extroversion being, judgmental or permissive or being compulsive or obsessive particularly with regard to food. Carefully and appropriately, the Personal Trainer asks questions with regard to family status, spouse relations, children's influence, family meals, etc. The initial Personal Trainer interview can be completed at one sitting, broken into convenient sessions, or self-administered by material provided via the internet. Its goal is to allow the Personal Trainer to "know" the client on an individual basis.

The initial visit should also include taking the patient's height, weight, blood pressure, and pulse. A log is kept, recording height once, weight at least once per week, blood pressure and pulse rate on a daily basis to chart progress. A scale that is consistent and accurate should be used, preferably before eating and drinking, and without clothing.

(Note: a physical examination by the family physician including an electrocardiogram is advisable on a yearly basis.)

With this information, the client is interviewed by the Personal Trainer, establishing the first real personal contact. During this initial interview, motivation is stressed, determination is reinforced, goals are tentatively set and the program is carefully explained.

The issue of food substitution is explained in detail. It is explained, based on the history obtained in the personal interview, in terms that are easily understood. It compares, for example, the program provision of food (carbohydrate, fat and protein) to the client's habitual intake of food as answered in the interview. A substitute meal (shake) is explained as to its constituent parts (low carbohydrate, no fat, percent of daily protein requirement, vitamins, antioxidants, and minerals). The client is reassured as to the safety and wholesomeness of the meal substitutes. He is given the wide choice of flavors and options of specific programs (Total, Moderate 2 + 2, or Moderate 3 + 1).

Appetite suppressants are explained in chemical and medical detail and an option is given for their use initially, later or not at all. Pharmaceuticals are left out of the initial interview to be determined later as to need. The pharmaceuticals currently used by the client have already been determined in the medical and personal histories. Nutriceuticals are then explained as to the reason for their use and the option of obtaining them from the Personal Trainer or elsewhere.

Finally, the conditions of physical activity are advised. It is stressed that exercise should be delayed for at least a week and then entered at a rate consistent with their renewed energy level and energy reserve.

When the initial Personal Trainer interview is complete, a specific program is selected to try for one to two weeks. The methods for contact, renewal of motivation and determination is specifically instructed, a means for obtaining the food substitutes appropriate to the program selected and the source of appetite suppressants is set. The same source of pharmaceuticals and nutriceuticals is instructed. A weekly log of physical activity is initiated.

The Personal Trainer Program has begun.

www.ingramcontent.com/pod-product-compliance
Lightning Source LLC
Chambersburg PA
CBHW060440290526
45793CB00002B/511